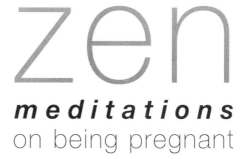

# zen

### *meditations*
## on being pregnant

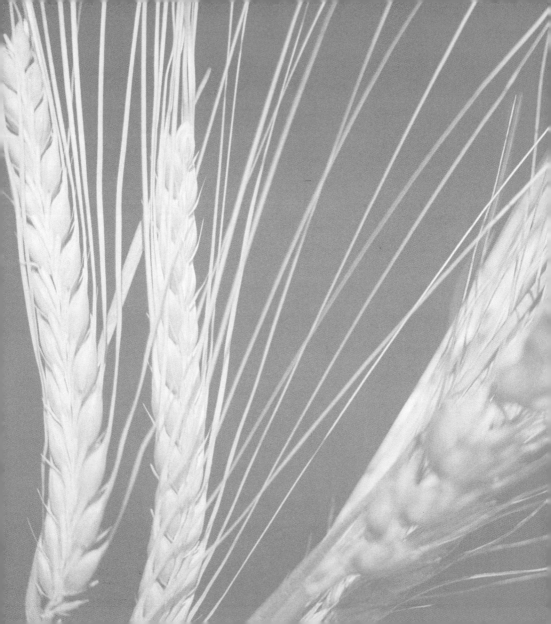

roni jay

# zen
*meditations*
on being pregnant

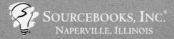

SOURCEBOOKS, INC.®
NAPERVILLE, ILLINOIS

Being pregnant is an exciting—sometimes frightening—journey into the unknown. It is a time of immense physical and emotional challenge when the thoughts naturally turn inward.

There are so many questions that cannot be answered simply: "Will the baby be OK?" "Will I cope with the birth?" "Will I cope after birth?" "Will I be a good parent?" No two women experience pregnancy in the same way, and advice from others can be as infuriating as it can be helpful. Only you can find your own way to deal with your experiences, take from others what is useful and positive, but leave behind that which worries you or makes you feel inadequate.

This may be your first baby, or you may already have children, you may be working outside the home—whatever your situation, pregnancy is a period of huge emotional demands. It is important at this time to make sure that you dedicate some time to yourself in which to try and think about, and deal with, some of the thoughts that are racing through your mind. This little book is designed to help you take a few moments to yourself to sit quietly and contemplate your pregnancy. Each meditation deals with a different aspect of being pregnant, the worries, the anticipation, the questions, and the excitement. It is both reassuring and wise, encouraging you to approach this time of great change with a calm and balanced attitude. To help you concentrate and wind down we have enclosed a CD of specially composed music which has been designed to create a soothing atmosphere. Listen to it while you meditate, or simply lie back and relax…

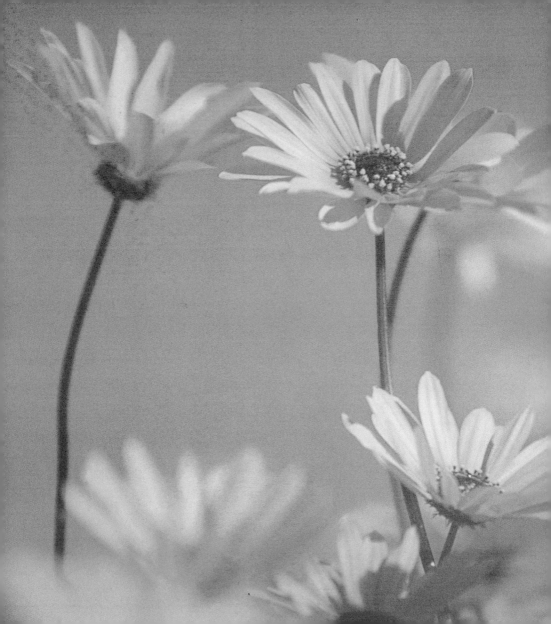

# birth and rebirth

Learning you are pregnant is like preparing for two births: your baby's, and your own rebirth. We know that we are entering a new phase of our life, so different from this phase that it is like a new life altogether. We are being reborn as a mother, and we cannot really know what it will be like until we arrive there. So the few months of pregnancy are a time to prepare for not one new life, but two.

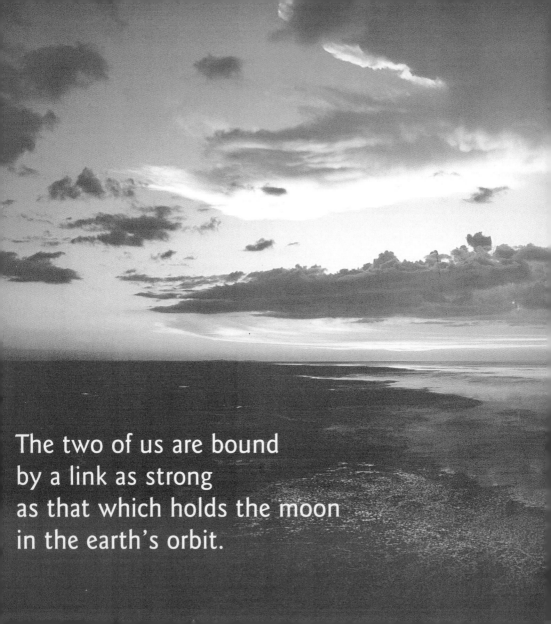

The two of us are bound
by a link as strong
as that which holds the moon
in the earth's orbit.

The moon is not a part of the earth, and yet
its movements are determined by the earth.
In return, it controls the earth's tides. In
the same way, our baby is not a part of us,
and yet its very existence, its health, its
growth are determined by us. And as it
grows within us, it influences our moods
and our physical comfort. The two of us are
bound by a link as strong as that which
holds the moon in the earth's orbit.

moon baby

# taking
# advice

The wise woman listens to everyone, but most of all to herself. When we are pregnant, everyone gives us advice. Every mother has learnt from her experience and wants to pass it on. All their advice is right—for themselves. But we are not them. Some of their advice will not work for us. So we can appreciate and listen to all they say, and then resolve to do it our own way. It is our pregnancy, our baby. Only we can know what is right for us. We may not have their experience of being pregnant, but they don't have our experience of being us.

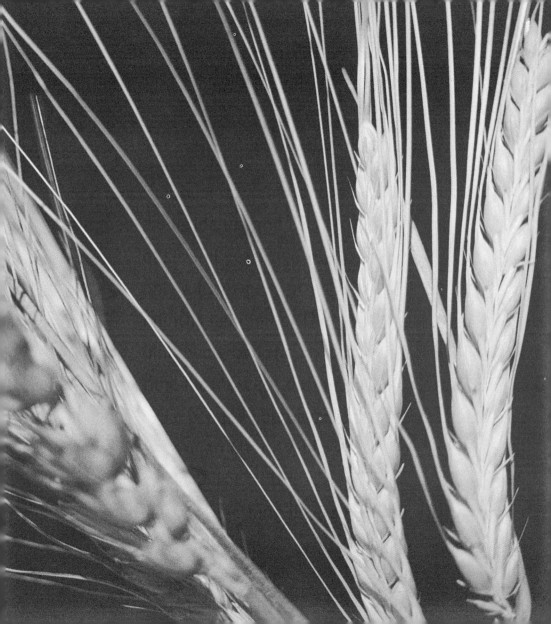

If you plant a rose bush, you first choose a spot
where it can thrive, then you feed the ground and
weed it, prepare the
soil for planting, and
water it ready for
the new rose. When

preparation

we are pregnant, those few months have a purpose.
They are preparation time, not only to buy bottles
and baby clothes, but also to prepare our world—
our new baby's world. Pregnancy is a time to plan
the kind of emotional world our child will grow up
in, the kind of things we will teach it, the ways we
will stimulate it, and how we will help it learn right
from wrong. They are a precious few months, and
not to be wasted.

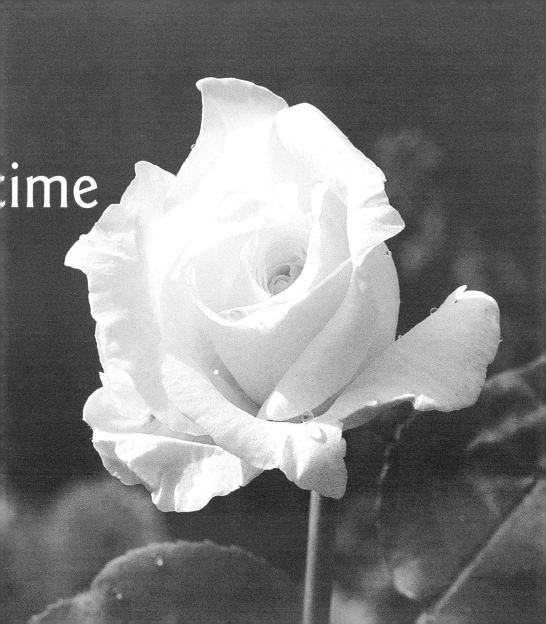

time

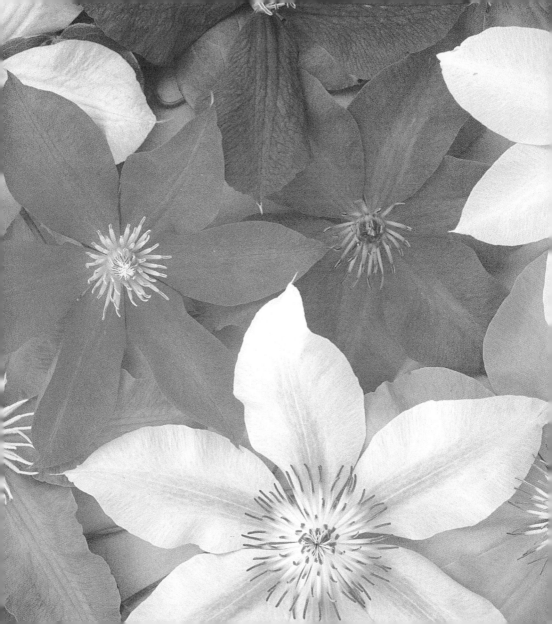

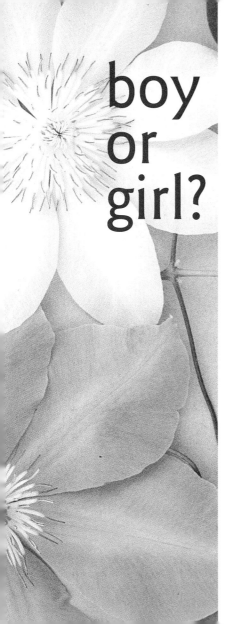

# boy or girl?

Every leaf on a tree is different; every pebble on the beach has its own shape and color; each snowflake is unlike any other. We focus on whether our baby will be a boy or a girl, but every boy is unique, and so is every girl. Our baby will be its own individual self whatever sex it is. We might as well question what kind of leaf, or pebble, or snowflake it will be— will it be even tempered or challenging, a joker or a serious thinker, a talker or a listener? All these things are equally interesting —and equally unanswerable for now—as the small matter of whether it will be a boy or a girl.

# worrying over nothing

When we make the decision to have a baby, we worry if it is the right decision. When we are carrying the child, we worry whether it will be healthy. As we near the end of the pregnancy, we worry whether labor will go well. And once the baby is born, we are set on a path of worrying for years. But all this worrying is human nature; as the child grows up we become more used to the worry, and more relaxed about it. But to worry at the start of the journey is simply a sign that the baby is important, and that we care. It is not a sign that there is anything wrong.

It is human
nature to worry
over the things
which matter
to us.

# what do we know?

## Does a bird on its nest know what baby bird will come out of each of the eggs it tends so carefully?

As an apple grows on the tree, does the tree know that the apple has seeds inside it? When a flower's seeds are ready to fall, does the flower know how tall the new flower springing from each seed will be? As we carry our baby inside us, we know almost nothing about it that distinguishes it from anyone else's baby—except that we love it unlike any other baby.

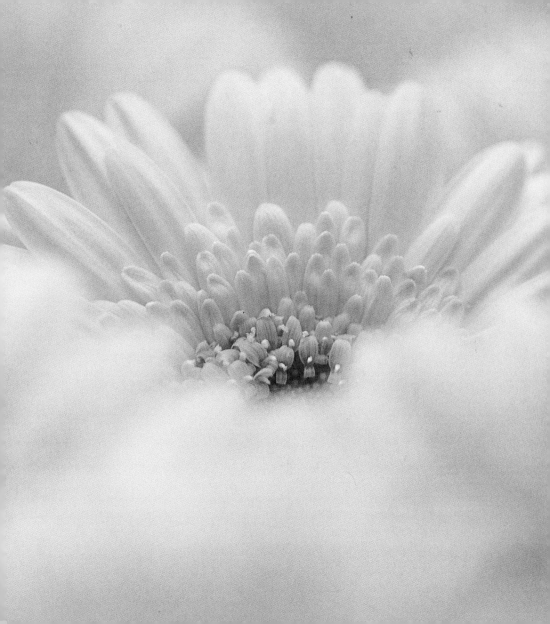

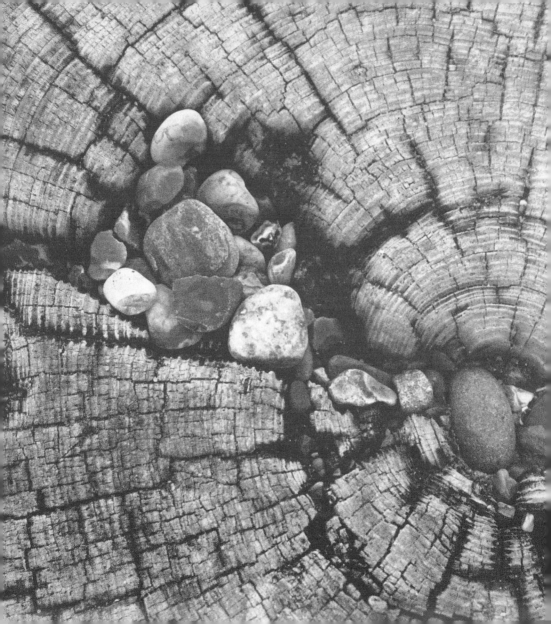

# feeling ill

When a tree drops a rotting branch, it does it for the best and improves the health of the rest of the tree. Some adult birds endure cold and hunger to sit on their eggs and keep them warm, knowing that it is worth it in the end. We may feel sick and unwell during pregnancy but we are not ill; we know it is a necessary part of the process. And in exchange for the discomfort of pregnancy, we will have a baby so beautiful that we willingly endure the sickness, the bad back, and the sleepless nights. They will all pass in a few months, but the baby will still be there when they are long gone.

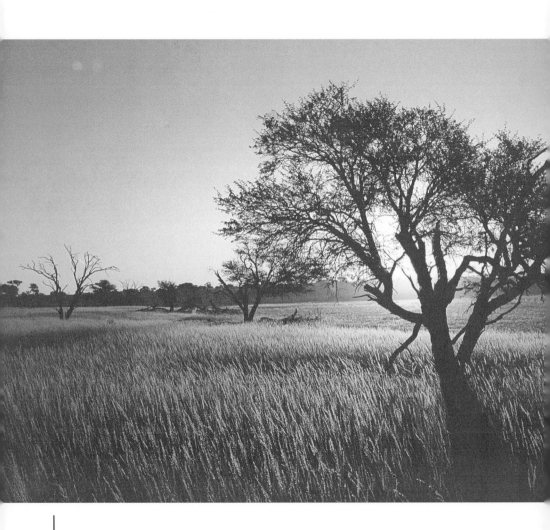

Time travels at a different speed at different times of our lives. As children, it appears to move so slowly it is unbearable at times, waiting for the holidays or the next birthday. But as we grow older, time speeds

# the passage of time

alongside us, and events of several years ago seem only a few weeks or months behind us. The older we grow, the faster time flies. Except during pregnancy. Being pregnant is like being a child again, those few months seeming to take an eternity, like a six-year-old waiting for a promised visit to the circus. Only this time, waiting for something bigger and better than ever before.

A sculptor can take a lump of wood, and create
something from it which the tree it came from would
be unable to recognize as its own—and yet that tree
is the first creator. In the same way, we and our
partner between us have sculpted something which
is made entirely from the two of us, and yet will
have a life and a form unique to itself.

# the art of creation

**It will be our baby, and yet it will
be in no one's image but its own.**

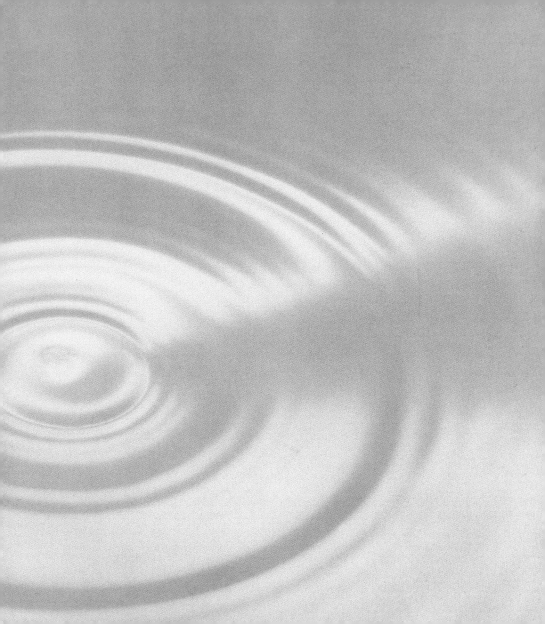

In the autumn, many animals are busy foraging for food, eating as much as they can before the long hibernation begins. It is not done with any resentment of hibernating; it is simply what happens. During our first pregnancy we can do many things we will find much harder once the baby arrives: waking late in the morning, going out for the evening, taking a long slow bath, reading the Sunday papers for hours. So why not enjoy them while we can? When we have fed our full on these pleasures, just as the mice and squirrels binge on nuts and berries, we will be happy to spend a few months or years with fewer late mornings, evenings out and Sunday papers.

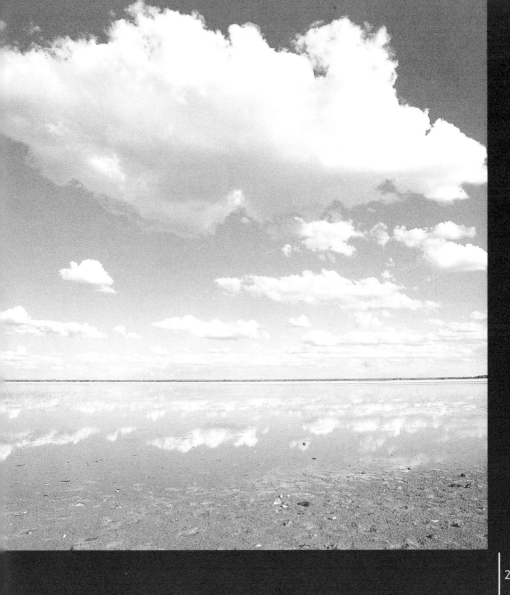

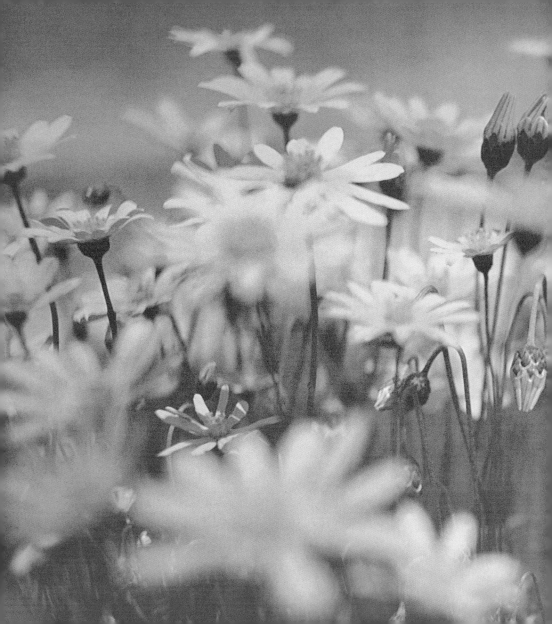

When a new garden is created, everyone takes credit for it. When an idea succeeds, many people lay claim to it. Once we announce we are pregnant, many people feel they have a stake in the baby, because they want to be a part of something wonderful. They touch our belly (without asking) to feel it kicking, they predict whether it will be a boy or a girl, they give us advice, they start knitting clothes. Some of this attention is welcome, some of it less so. But it is done because everyone can see that we are doing something magical, and they want a little piece of the magic to spill over onto them.

# whose baby?

# weak or strong?

An unborn baby seems almost unimaginably weak and vulnerable, like a feather in a typhoon, or a flower at the summit of a volcano that is about to erupt. And yet babies are designed to survive with a strength and endurance which is extraordinary. And we are part of their strength, with our instinct to put our hands over our belly, or to keep our stomach protected if we happen to fall. With our help the baby

—however frail it feels—has
the strength to face the
journey from a single cell
to a human being.

The bond which links the earth to the sun is invisible and intangible, but it is no less strong for that. And the bond which links us to our unborn baby is far stronger than the umbilical cord which forms the physical link. It is a bond which

# bonding

often forms in our own heart before the baby is even conceived, and strengthens every day even after the child is born. And it is a bond which will last for as long as the earth continues to circle the sun.

When you see the shape of an animal in a piece of driftwood, it becomes that animal. When you are treated like a queen, you feel like a queen. When we are pregnant, strangers in the street defer to us, we are offered a seat, served first, invited to put our feet up. We are treated like royalty. And because we are regarded as being special, we feel special. And so we should. We are doing the most special thing anyone can: bringing new life into the world.

Let's enjoy feeling like a queen while we know we deserve it.

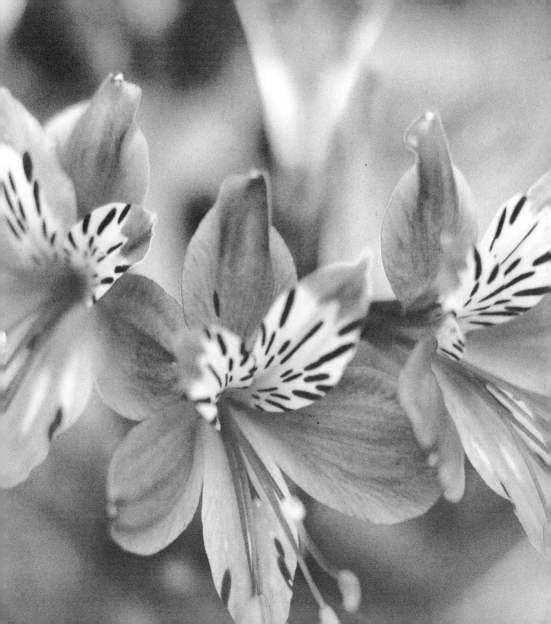

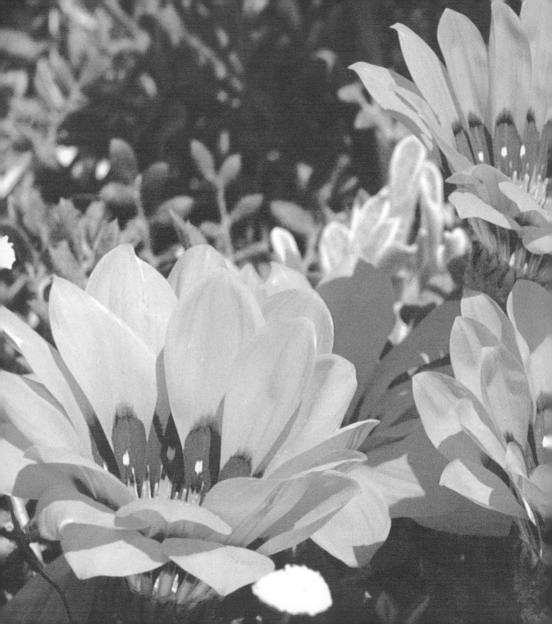

# seeing
# the best
# of people

Pregnancy is a blessing in many ways; one of its blessings is that it brings out the best in people. People who have never met us feel they can talk to us, share their own experience of pregnancy and babies with us, wish us luck. Passers-by smile at us, strangers hold doors open for us. Pregnancy is a blessed state because we see a side of human nature which is positive and good. A side of human nature we want our baby to grow up with.

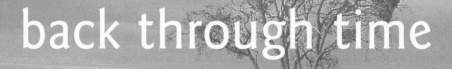

# back through time

**Every oak tree grows from an acorn which fell from another oak,**

which itself grew from an acorn from yet another oak tree. When we give birth to our first child, we begin a new generation. We add the next link in a chain which reaches back past our mother and our grandmothers, to our great-grandmothers, and our great-great-grandmothers, and beyond. The chain we are helping to forge has seen the 20th century, the Industrial Revolution, the Middle Ages, the Roman Empire and more. We and our baby are the links which will extend the chain forward through our grandchildren and great-grandchildren, and on to who knows what?

# be selfish

When you have a secret, you can savor and relish it, and enjoy keeping it to yourself. But once you tell others it becomes a shared thing, no longer your secret. A pregnancy may be no secret, but while the baby is inside us, we can relish and enjoy keeping it to ourselves. Once it is born, others will want to hold it and play with it, rock it to sleep, or feed it. Only for now can we keep it all to ourselves for a few precious months, and no one can expect us to share.

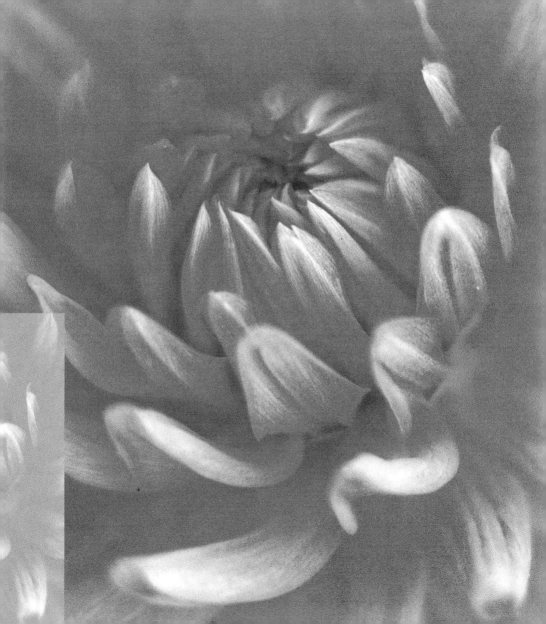

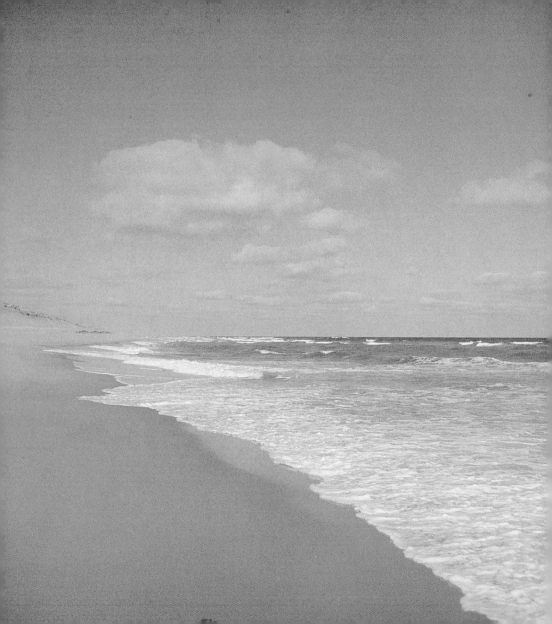

# greater than the sum

If you take a seed and give it water and sunlight, you create something which is far more than merely seed, water and sunshine. You create new life. Something which is greater than the sum of its parts.

In the same way, we are the same person we always were, but add a baby and we create something greater than both. We create not only life but also a new focus of love, a new relationship, a new inspiration for us, the baby, and those around us. Together with our baby, we become greater than the sum of our parts.

When a tree produces fruit, it
puts its strength into creating the
best fruit it can, containing strong
seed to grow into a new tree. Even
though the leaves on an apple tree
may be blighted and some of its
branches dying, the apples are
shiny and healthy, and bursting
with seeds. Our bodies are the
same. They cream off the best of
everything and give it to the baby.
We may feel tired and aching,

# putting your baby

but still our body makes sure
that the baby has everything
it needs to thrive. And would we want it any other way?

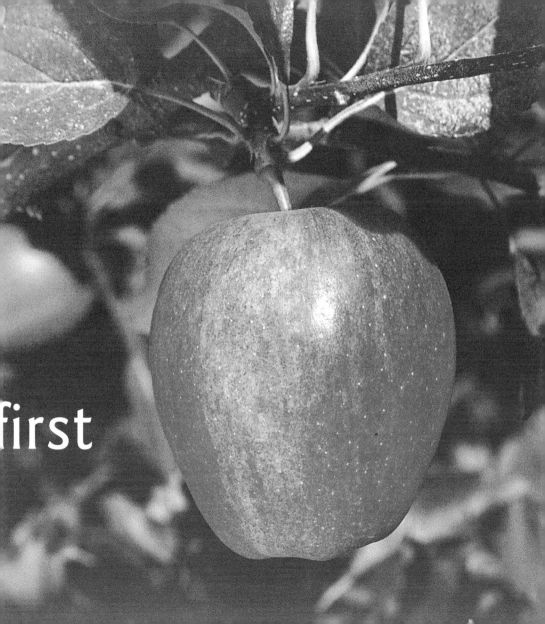

first

# not alone

Like an apprentice who is not trusted to cope alone, our partners must stand on the sidelines and watch as we take center stage. We are the lucky ones, carrying the baby. We may joke about how men would feel if they had to do it, but many men envy our closeness to the baby, and our involvment. And even when we complain of the tiredness, and the aches and pains, most of us would be reluctant to give it all up and watch our partner hold the baby in our place, and form the bond that we now have. Would we not be envious then?

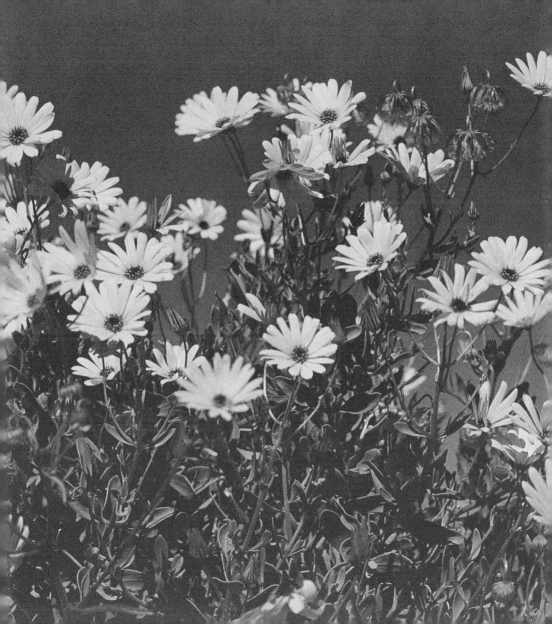

greater love

Many of the
smallest creatures of
the earth care for and
tend their babies.
Sparrows, mice, even
scorpions look after
their little ones. So we,
with our understanding,
our lifelong bond with
our children, our ability
to contemplate the
future—surely we must
be capable of greater
love for the child inside
us than any other
creature on earth.

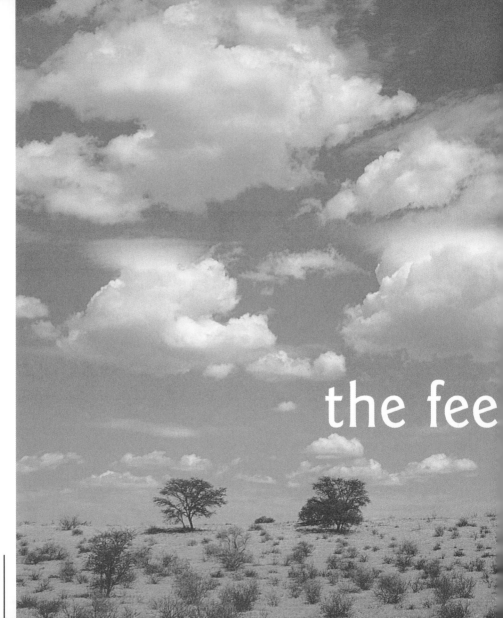

the fee

The message of a
hilltop beacon, or
smoke rings on
the horizon, is
not complex but
it is very clear.

Communication does not have to be detailed to be
important. And the first kicking of a baby inside us

**of feet**

is our first direct communication
with our new child. We can feel it
respond to our movements, and we
reply with a stroke or a soft word.

Those first movements may feel as gentle as a
butterfly's wings, but they are a blazing beacon to us.

As a pebble
on the beach
is slowly
worn down
by the sea,
it sits patiently, and each day it is minutely smoother than it
was yesterday. Our pregnancy might seem to last for ever,
but each day is different. Each day the child within is being
gradually shaped, like the pebble. If we wish the pregnancy
over with, we wish
away all those precious            patience
moments of our baby's
life. However far ahead
the pregnancy stretches, never after today will we be exactly
twenty weeks pregnant with this child, or thirty-three
weeks, or whatever it is. If we are patient, like the pebble on
the beach, we will enjoy each day for itself and the moment
                                          of birth will
                                          still arrive
                                          when it is
                                          ready.

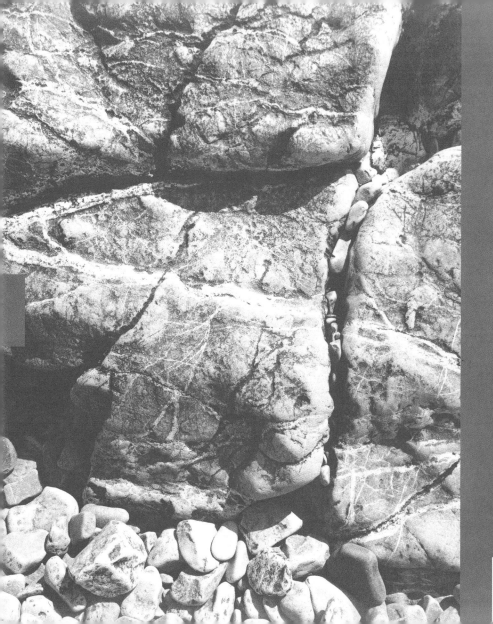

The purpose of a lion is to have cubs.
The purpose of a butterfly is to lay eggs.
The purpose of a fruit tree is to bear fruit.
And the purpose of humans is to bear children.

created

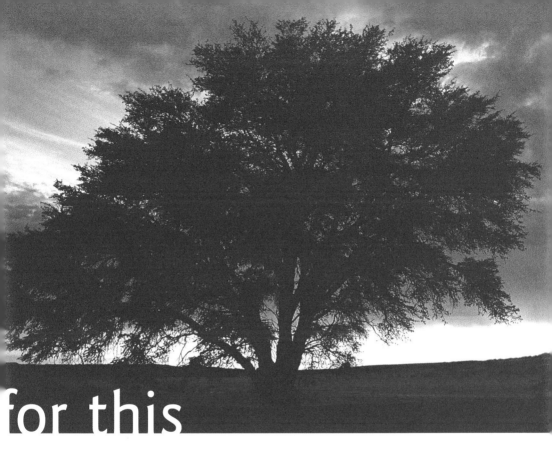

## for this

Every living thing has, as its ultimate purpose, the perpetuation of the species. When we become pregnant, we become part of a natural cycle which links us to every other living plant and animal on the planet. We share the same goal as the lion, the butterfly, and the fruit tree.

# helping the bigger ones

Even a tiger prowls cautiously in unknown territory. When we don't know what to expect we are often nervous, even frightened. We know that nothing can fully prepare us for the impact of a new baby, but— if we have done it before—we have at least some idea. How much more unprepared our other children must be for the changes a new brother or sister will bring.

**Even the bravest, most tiger-like child will be fearful inside.**

The piping of a flute can charm a snake; a plant will grow taller if it grows to the sound of music. And a baby, too, will respond to sounds even before it is born. We are responsible for the sounds our baby hears while we carry it. We can choose whether it hears the sound of traffic, birdsong, television, singing, its parents arguing, crowds, or music. Of course we don't have a choice twenty-four hours a day, but we do have a choice much of the time—time enough to create a prevailing mood. We can put on gentle music when we get home from work, sing to it while we drive the car, talk softly to it when we say goodnight.

If a lethally poisonous snake can be tamed with

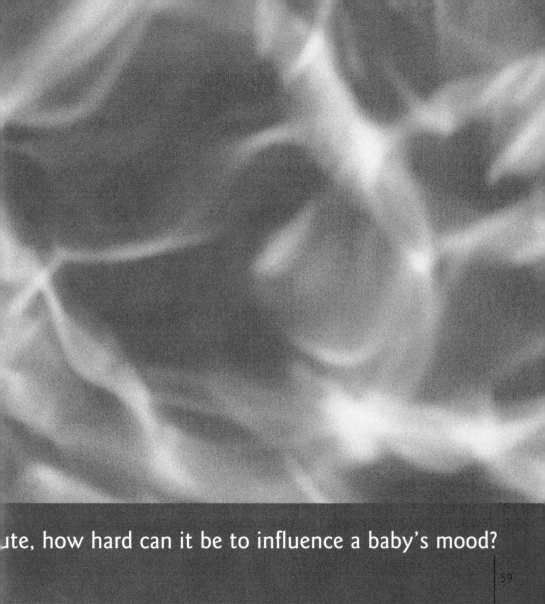

ute, how hard can it be to influence a baby's mood?

# once upon a time...

A great river starts as a trickling stream; the tallest tree begins as a tiny shoot; the biggest city was once only a little village. From presidents and monarchs to humble workers, we all began life as a few cells clustered together and beginning to grow into life. The child we carry inside is following the path we have all followed before. Even we were once held tight and safe inside our own mother's womb, just as our baby is now. And our mother felt the same bond with us that we now feel with our own child. We may not be able to imagine our baby's life inside the womb, but we have lived it.

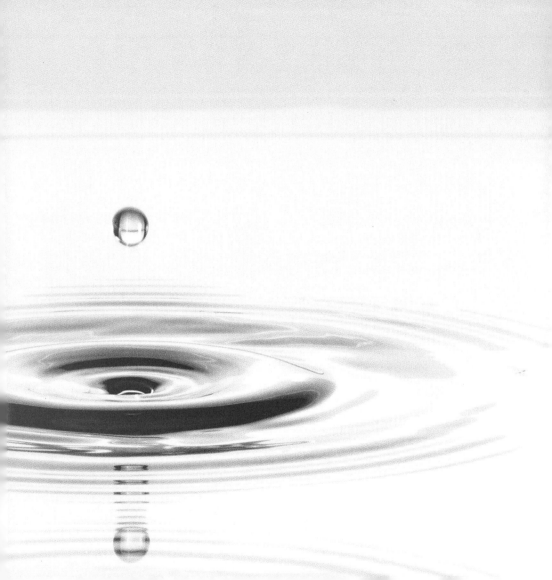

in the beginning

As we set out upon an unknown road, with no map, we cannot know where it will lead us. We know only that it will be a long journey with many adventures along the way. The first few steps seem hugely significant, but they are a tiny fraction of the whole. The journey from conception to birth seems long and full of mystery, but it is only the first of many, many stages on the journey. Alongside our child, we will travel further than we can imagine now, and these first few steps will seem very distant indeed before we reach the end of our road together.

On an overcast day, the sun is hidden from us behind a blanket of clouds. Yet when the clouds part and the sun shines brightly down, we are not surprised to see it. We knew it was there all along,

# celebrating the day

just waiting for a break in the clouds. It is the same when the baby is born. Others may say "A new baby!" but to us, the baby has been sentient and full of life for months. It has simply waited until now to appear. The date of its birth may be important to others, but to us it doesn't mark the beginning of new life, only the moment when the sun broke through the clouds.

of birth

# chill out

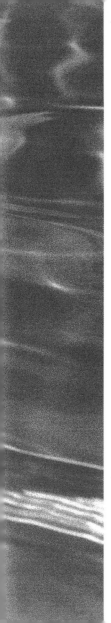

A stone falling into a still pool makes the
water ripple. Whatever we do has an
effect around us; we cannot operate in
isolation. This is increased even more
when it is the baby inside us—linked to us
both physically and emotionally—that is
affected. If we allow ourselves to become
stressed, we are passing that stress on to our
child. Of course we cannot help being
stressed from time to time, but we owe it to
our baby as well as ourselves to be as happy
and relaxed as we can be. Instead of dropping
a stone into the pool, how much better to
ripple the water with a gentle breeze, or a
beautiful leaf floating lightly on the surface.

fear

# of change

A bear cub hibernating for its first winter has no idea what spring will be like. A caterpillar wrapped in its cocoon doesn't yet understand how it feels to fly. And, as we carry our first baby inside us, we have no real conception of the change it will bring to our lives. We hear people tell us "life will never be the same again" and "you don't know what you're in for," and it is easy to fear the future. But change, when it comes, can be wonderful; it doesn't have to be intimidating.

The young bear cub welcomes the spring joyfully, and how could the caterpillar not be happy to take to the air and fly?

Our partner has an equal stake in the baby, and an equal responsibility for it. We may be doing the work for now, but they will be doing their share soon enough. They have as many fears and worries as we do, not least the fear of losing us. Lovemaking has many benefits, physical, mental, emotional and spiritual. During pregnancy, we both need the emotional reassurance of lovemaking. It

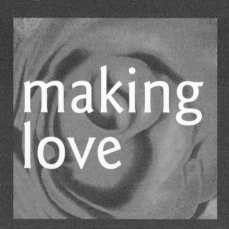

## making love

may not always be as physically adventurous as it was, but it can be emotionally deeper and more exciting than ever before.

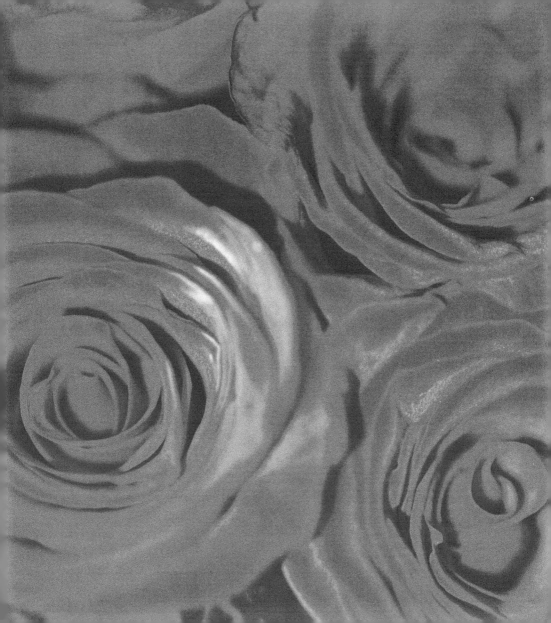

# the grand scheme

Is there
a God?
How can
something
as complex
and intricate
as our world
be created
by chance?

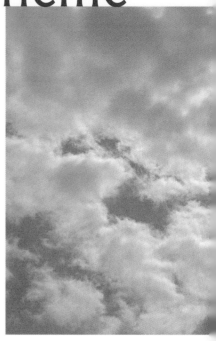

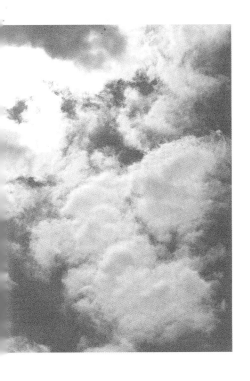

Whatever our religious or spiritual beliefs, pregnancy is a time when it seems clear that there is a great pattern, repeating through our lives and those that have gone before, and will come after. Whatever force created the pattern, it seems inconceivable that it could be purely random. We are taking our place, with our baby, in the grand scheme of things.

# bad dreams

Some people predict the future from tea leaves left in the cup. And down the ages dreams have been considered an indication of what is to come. But dreams have many functions. They help us come to terms with worries, fears, and preoccupations, so we naturally dream of our fears about our baby or about labor. During pregnancy we sleep more lightly than usual, so we both dream more, and remember more of our dreams, including more of the bad ones. But these pregnancy nightmares are no bad omen; they are simply helping our unconscious mind prepare for the transition to motherhood.

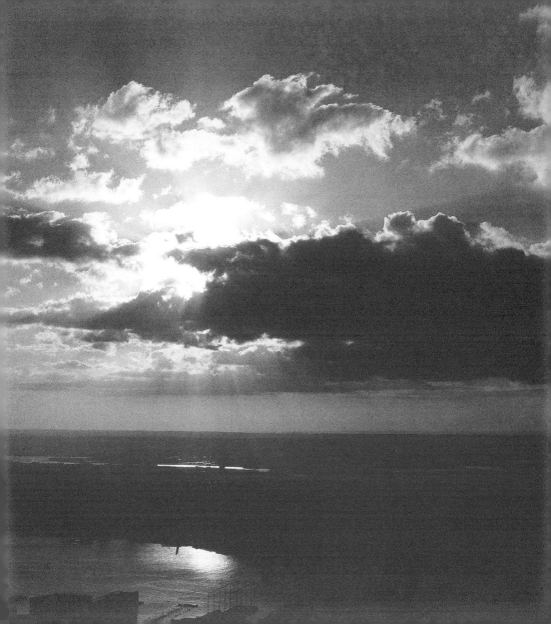

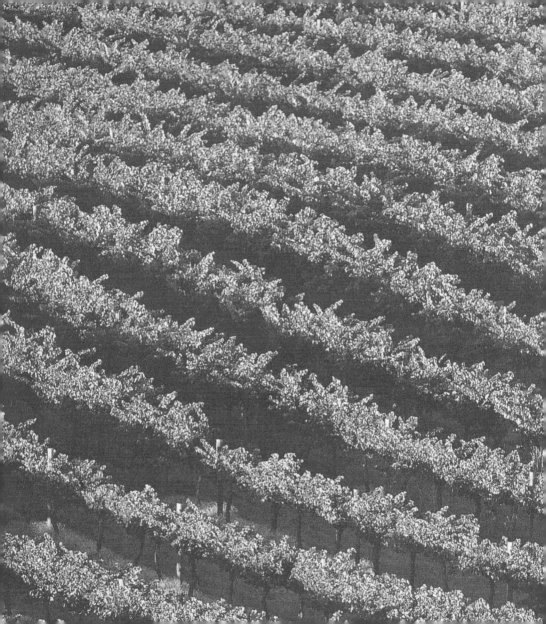

When a pair of oxen draw a plough, both must work in unison. For us to work together with our partner to bring up our baby, we too must work as a team.

# teamwork

Part of the preparation of pregnancy is learning to work in unison with our partner. Without children, we may have managed fine as a couple without needing to be a real team. Once the baby arrives, true teamwork will be crucial. This is our time to plan and practice so that, like the oxen, we can plough a strong, straight furrow.

# size isn't everything

We live in a culture where thin is best. As women, there is a great pressure to watch our weight, and preserve our figure. Pregnancy goes against all this. As the baby starts to show, we may know the reason, but to most people we simply look overweight. But we have something far more important than a slim profile, and soon enough it will be too clear to mistake for mere extra bodyweight. The prospect of a new life puts such petty concerns into perspective.

## Which would we rather have: a fla

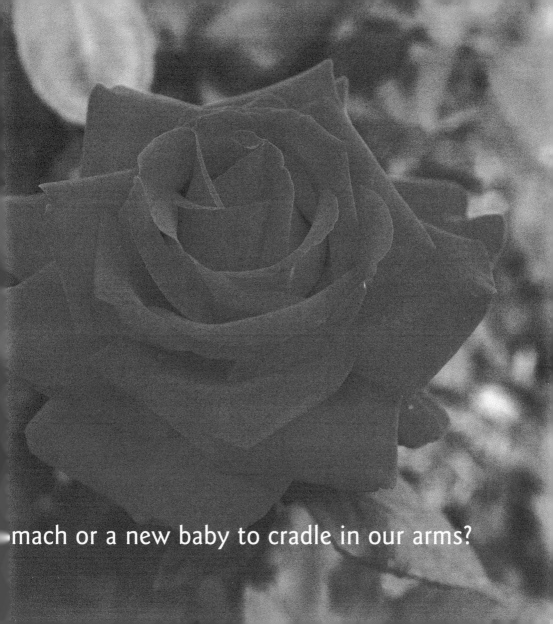

mach or a new baby to cradle in our arms?

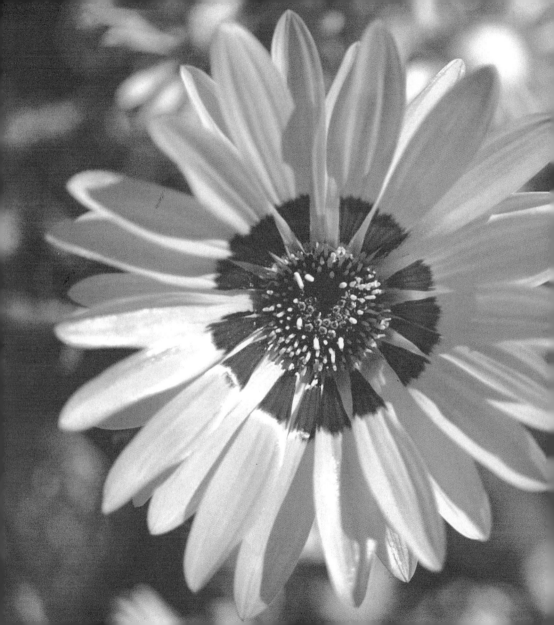

When champions win a race, they take a lap of honor. When performers win an award, they make an acceptance speech. How much more do we deserve praise, for creating, nurturing and carrying a new life within us? We are entitled to carry our pregnancy with pride; it is worth all the laps of honor and silver trophies that others receive for far lesser achievements.

# wear it with pride

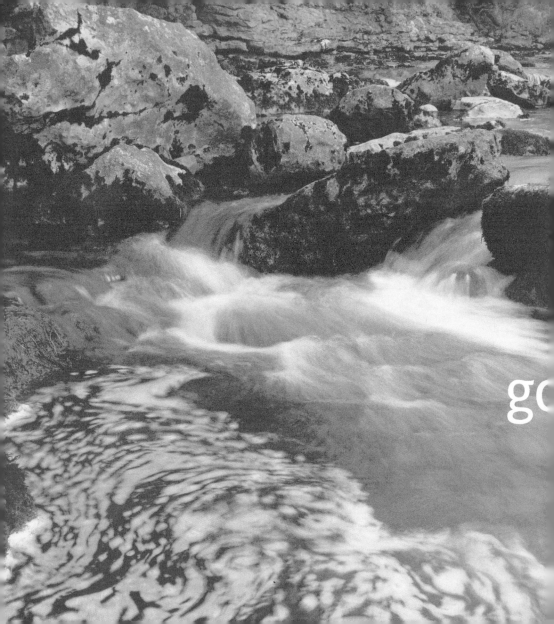

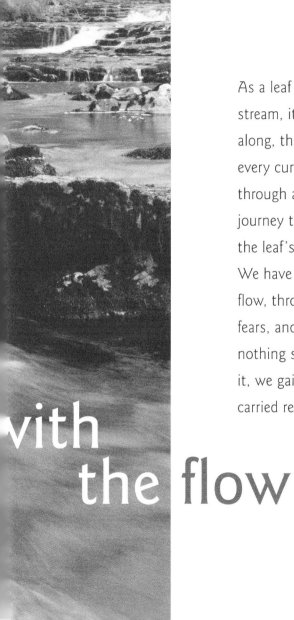

As a leaf spins on the surface of a stream, it allows itself to be carried along, through all the eddies and on every current, down waterfalls and through almost still, deep pools. Our journey through our pregnancy is like the leaf's journey down the stream. We have no choice but to go with the flow, through the worries and the fears, and the still, deep pools where nothing seems to progress. If we fight it, we gain nothing—we will still be carried remorselessly downstream.

with the flow

A bird in springtime gathers up twigs and feathers to prepare a nest to lay its eggs in. When we buy or borrow strollers and cribs, blankets and mobiles, we are following the same instinct. A crib is not only a comfortable bed to sleep in, it will also represent security for our child. A car seat will keep it safe, and toys will give it vital mental stimulation. Our nest may be bigger and more elaborate than the birds', but it is no less important. The process of creating it is necessary, on both a practical and an emotional level, and we should relax and enjoy it.

# getting ready

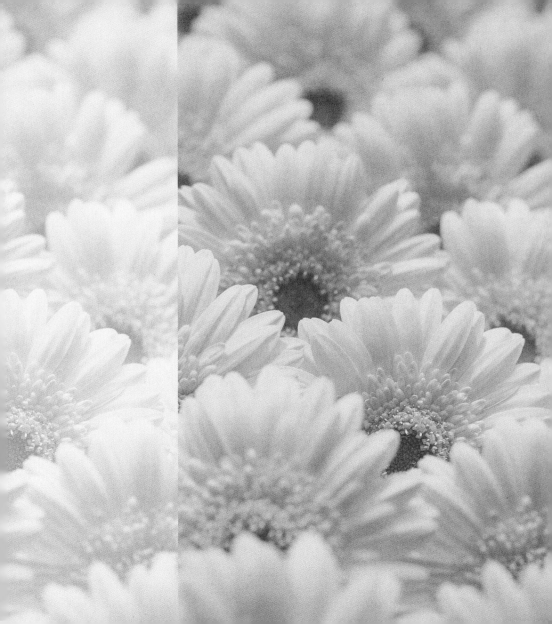

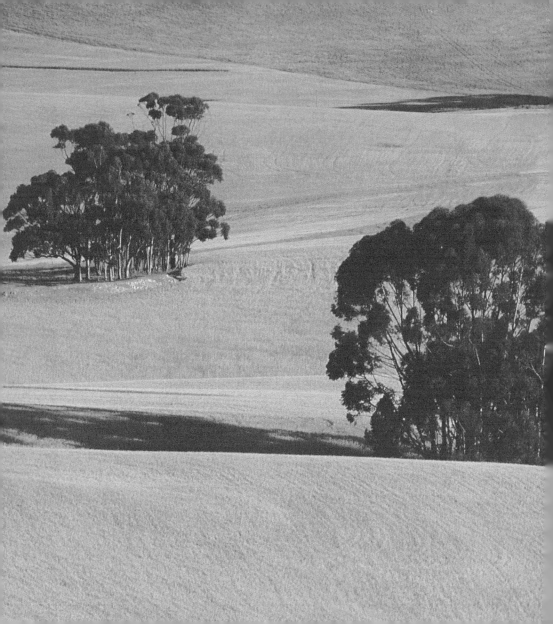

# enduring
# the waiting

In the Arctic, the long winter seems to last
almost forever before spring finally arrives.
In arid tropical regions, the dry season drags
by for most of the year until the rains finally
come. Waiting for the birth, especially if it is
late, can seem similar. We grow heavier and
more uncomfortable, we are anxious to see
our baby and to begin our new life with it,
and everything just seems to stand still. We
can only try to enjoy our last few days or
weeks of free time, knowing that however
far off it seems, the spring will come at last.

## beyond imagination

If you have never stood on top of a mountain, you cannot really know how it feels. If you have never parachuted from a plane, you don't know what it is really like. It doesn't matter how eloquently a deep sea diver explains the feeling of being at the bottom of the ocean, you'd have to do it yourself to understand fully. And the same is true of childbirth. Throughout pregnancy we try to imagine it, but it cannot be described. The mix of physical, emotional, mental, and spiritual feelings is so complex, and so unique to each mother, that it can be understood only by experiencing it. So although we continue to wonder about it, we should not expect an answer until the moment itself arrives.

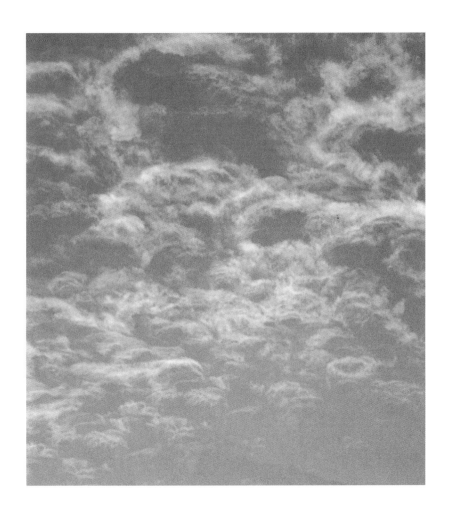

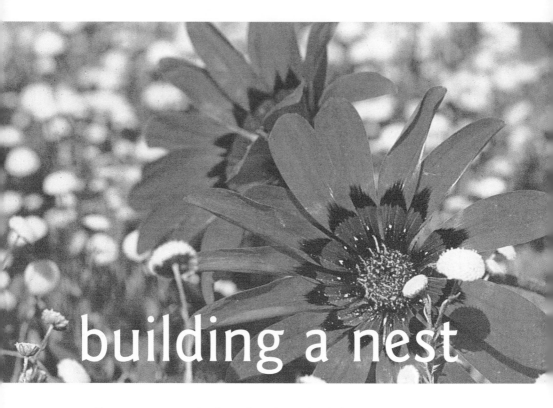

# building a nest

All parents want the best for their child, from the day it is born. And we are keen to start building a nest for it to grow up in before it has even arrived. So we decorate the nursery in the way we think best. Will it want bright shades or restful ones? Should we create a fantasy world of clouds and castles, or an

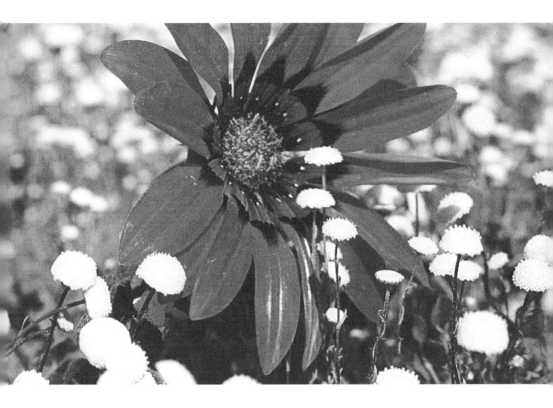

earthy world of elephants and giraffes? Or perhaps just clean, simple, plain colors? Even a basic question of whether we prefer orange or green will affect our baby. The choices we make now will contribute to our child's growing consciousness, so we need to be happy with them.

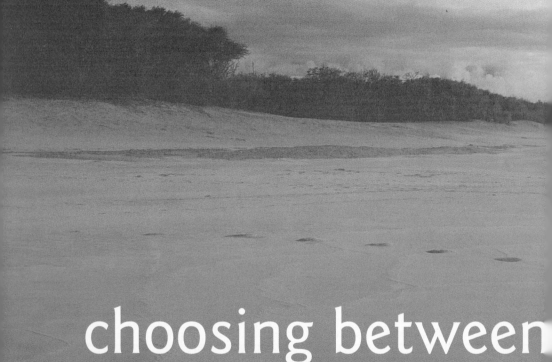

If we come to a fork in the road
in unknown territory, how can w

choosing between

We have no conception of what childbirth will be like, and yet friends and midwives ask us what kind of birth we want to have. How can we know? All we can do is decide which road looks most inviting, and start down that path. But we may need to cut across to some other route if the way is thornier than we expected. Better to plan only the road we will start on, and be ready for anything, than to decide the whole route in advance without having walked it before.

# unknowns

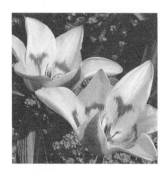
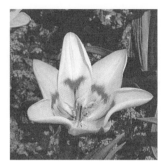
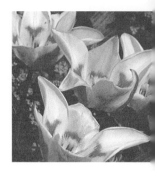
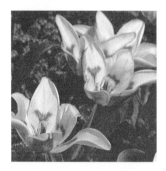

# right
## or
# wrong

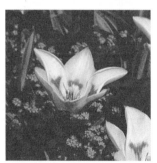
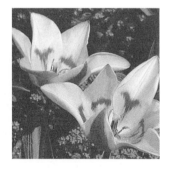
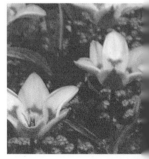

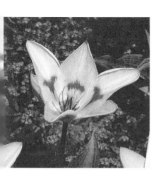

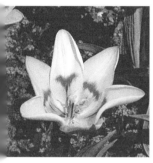

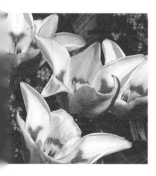

No one presumes to tell a mother bird that she is letting her fledglings fly the nest too early. No one tells the rose that it is wrong to flower in June. And yet many people tell us that pain relief in childbirth is wrong, that we ought to breastfeed our baby, that we shouldn't give birth at home. There is no right or wrong way to give birth. Pain relief may not be ideal, but nor is a distraught mother. Breast milk may be more nutritious than bottle milk, but both are satisfying for a hungry baby.

All that matters is that we choose what seems best, and make our choices for our baby with love.

# standing by

Every theatrical production needs a team of people to make it run smoothly. And the same holds true for producing a child. Our role in the birth is clear, along with the baby's. The nurses and midwives each have their part to play, too. But what of our partner? This is the birth of his child too, and he needs to feel included. We may be center stage, but he deserves at least a supporting role. If we write him a key part, his performance can make our role easier and we will all be involved, working toward the same first night première together.

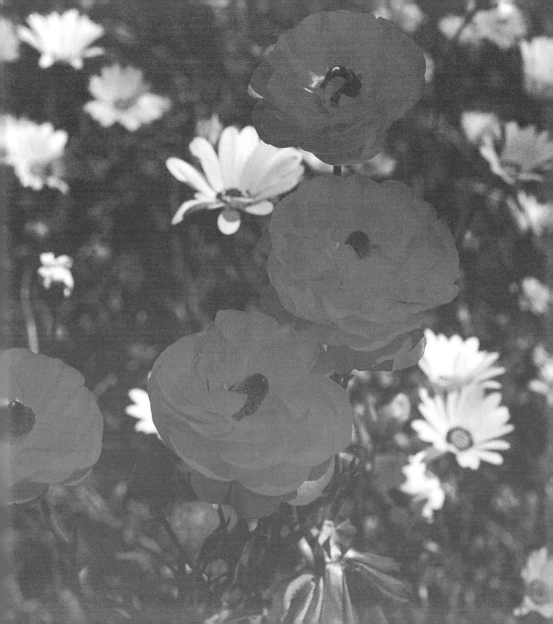

new
mother

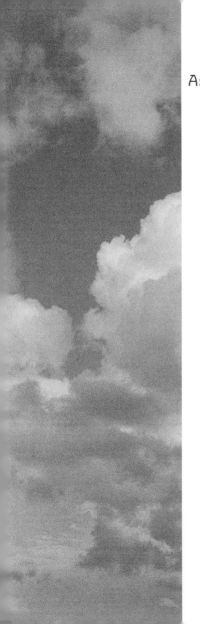

As a caterpillar metamorphoses into a butterfly, it turns into a new creature altogether. We go into labor as one person, but emerge as another. And for the rest of our life we will be this new creature—a mother. We have been a child, a teenager, a single person, a partner, but all of these have merged gradually one into another over time. We go from this life into motherhood in a matter of hours, and yet it is the greatest change of all.

Old soldiers who have fought in battle side by side talk of a deep bond of experience that others cannot share. Mothers speak of their bond less often, but they are just as aware of it.

# shared experience

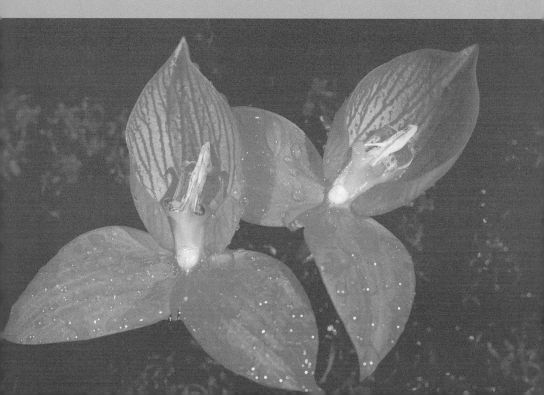

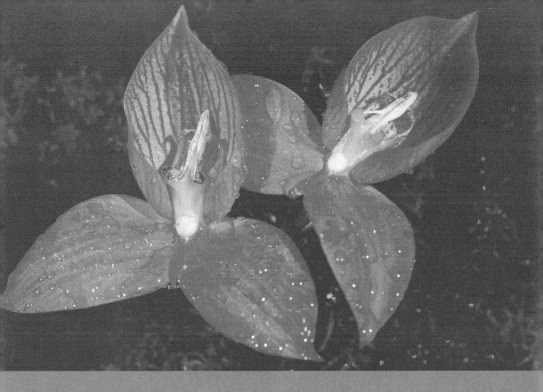

When other women see that we are pregnant, they smile or wink to acknowledge that shared experience—we are now part of a special group. Friends with children talk to us in a new way, knowing that we now understand—or soon will—a wealth of emotions and experiences which friends without children cannot know. We may never before have recognized the partnership mothers share, but once we join their ranks we are instantly aware of the bond.

# pain

Pain does not have to be
bad. Marathon runners
choose to put themselves
through immense pain to achieve
the winning post. Mountaineers
choose to endure great cold and
hardship to reach the summit. The
pain of childbirth is a good pain, a pain
that is meant to be. Some of us find it
easy to bear, others find it hard. But for all
of us it is part of the experience whether we
like it or not, and therefore part of something
which is, essentially, wonderful.

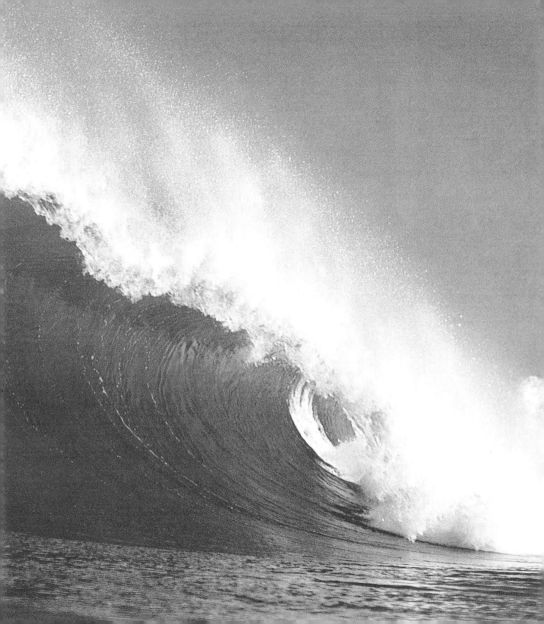

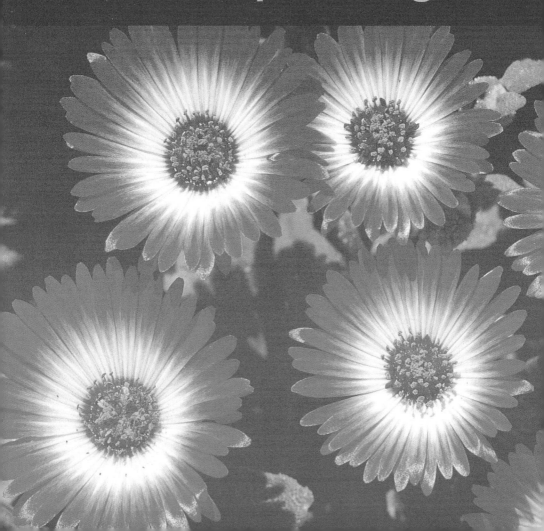

expanding love

When we love someone, we do not have to deny love to anyone else.

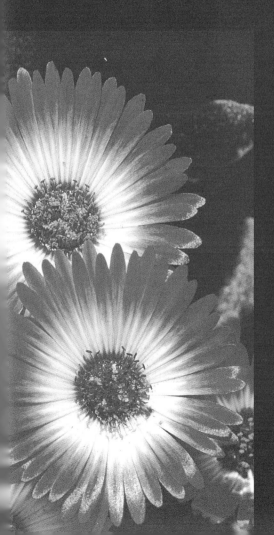

Rather, we increase our capacity to love. When we bring a baby into the world, we increase the love that we feel, and that everyone who ever loves our child throughout its life will feel. And we have created a new person with their own capacity to love, too. By giving birth, we have expanded the world's total store of love.

# Love is not finite.

# news

The moment the sun breaks over the horizon, the sky bursts into the colors of the dawn with the promise of a brand new day ahead. The moment at which the pregnancy is confirmed— whether by a doctor or by a thin blue line—is just such an outburst of color.

A new daw

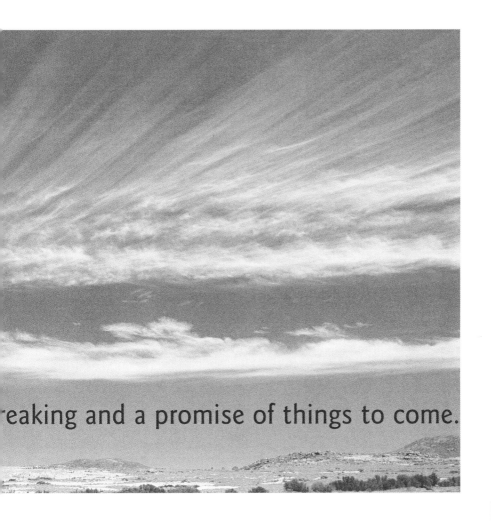

...eaking and a promise of things to come.

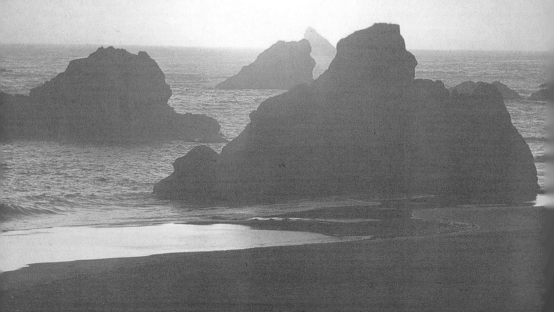

bond
of
love

The bond of love is even stronger than the physical cord which binds us to our child. Our feelings are transmitted to our growing baby along with all the other nourishment our body passes on. The baby will feel happy and secure when we simply think about how much we love it, and will always love it. A private, whispered message of love is as nourishing for us as it is for our baby.

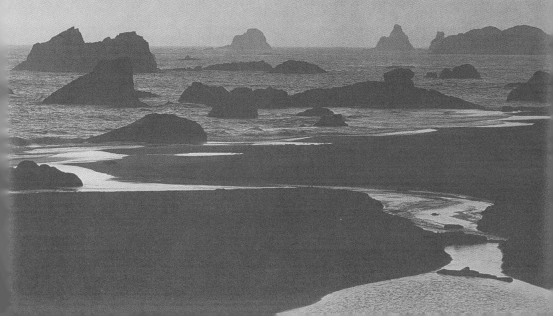

Sourcebooks, Inc.
P.O. Box 4410, Naperville, Illinois 60567-4410
(630) 961-3900
FAX: (630) 961-2168

Text © Roni Jay 2000
Cover design: The Big Idea
Interior design: Susannah Good
Cover image: Gill Orsman, Flowers & Foliage
Interior images: © Digital Vision
Series Editor: Elizabeth Carr

Printed in Italy

MQ 10 9 8 7 6 5 4 3 2 1

ISBN: 1-57071-644-7

## Note on the CD

The music that accompanies this book has been specially commissioned from composer David Baird. Trained in music and drama in Wales, and on the staff of the Welsh National Opera & Drama company, David has composed many soundtracks for both the theater and radio.

The CD can be played quietly through headphones while relaxing or meditating on the text. Alternatively, lie on the floor between two speakers placed at equal distances from you. Try and center your thoughts, and allow the soundtrack to wash over you and strip away the distracting layers of the outside world.